THE WAY OF THE CROSS FOR NURSES

By Ellen Rice

FOREWORD

I write these books to express my thoughts, but not to preach. As time goes on, I truly believe with St. Paul that I might be the worst of sinners. Not so much for what I have done, but for that which I could have done, and did not do.

So, I write… not because of who I am, but because I can articulate these ideas well. And because I can do so, I must do so.

I write the books I would like to read.

Let others, who are perfect, write the books that are perfect.

Ellen Rice, RN BSN

DEDICATION

To John

PREFACE

Graduates of Catholic schools will remember the Lenten Friday ritual of attending the Stations of the Cross. We adore you, O Christ, and we praise you. Because by your holy Cross you have redeemed the world.

The Stations of the Cross were a Western adaptation of the Via Dolorosa that pilgrims to Jerusalem would walk in the footsteps of Christ. When churches began including fourteen stations based on the Via Dolorosa, the Christian could take a virtual pilgrimage that many of them would not be able to take in their lifetime. In time, a fifteenth station was added, to commemorate the Resurrection, which reminds us that death and pain are never the end of the story.

For nurses, the Via Dolorosa, the road from the praetorium to Calvary hill is a metaphor for our daily walk through the units and community offices where we serve. Our sufferings and the sufferings of others mark this daily path; yet the final "station," the Resurrection, is entwined with the hope and boundless joy that we find in each day.

Alexander Solzhenitsyn once famously said that in the West we had Christ without the Cross, whereas in the Soviet Union they had the Cross without Christ.

Nursing, by its very nature, often brings us to the cross without Christ, with a side of life that can seem cruel and meaningless without a strong faith. Using His Cross to bring meaning to suffering is critical, lest we become lost amidst the intrinsic brutality of human pain and sorrow.

The Way of the Cross may be unfamiliar to Christians from Reformation traditions. It is a way of remembering Jesus's footsteps, a way of coping with the suffering of life by identifying it with our Redeemer. Although the Way of the Cross is a traditionally Catholic devotion, this booklet is intended for a wider Christian audience, as well as an audience amongst nurses of all faiths.

This devotional book of meditations is meant to help all nurses focus on the meaning behind the suffering that is part of their daily walk.

Each traditional station is named, and the traditional antiphon is included to focus our worship of Jesus, and our gratitude for the Cross. A meditation follows. Faith in action questions guide our own footsteps.

THE FIRST STATION: JESUS IS CONDEMNED TO DEATH

We adore you O Christ, and we praise you.

Because by your holy Cross, you have redeemed the world.

Our lives as nurses are filled with reminders of mortality. We do not worship suffering or mortality. Rather, we seek to glorify God by proclaiming His resurrection power. We alleviate suffering, we fight for life. When death comes at last, we seek to ease suffering and prepare the beloved to meet the Savior.

Jesus told us that whatever we do to the least of our brethren we do to Him. Collectively, those whom individuals or society causes suffering are identified with Jesus.

In nursing, we come across people every day who have been condemned. Poverty limits food choices and increases stress. Low birth weight and prematurity create adverse growth patterns and predict psychological issues.

Nursing shortages condemn patients to substandard care. In some corners of the world, medication shortages condemn people to death.

We are called to be Jesus' hands and feet today.

Faith in action

My professional life is only as good as my personal life. Nursing as it as currently envisioned demands "sacrifices" and often other people pay the price.

What person or people have I unjustly condemned to an adverse outcome by putting them second?

Can I see the face of Christ in the ignored friend, parent, brother or significant other?

How can I begin to make it up to them today… to be a nurse and neighbor for the nearest first and the patients second?

THE SECOND STATION: JESUS TAKES UP HIS CROSS

We adore you O Christ, and we praise you.

Because by your holy Cross, you have redeemed the world.

Can you even imagine being a god? Human history worshiped deities who lived on mountain tops or rode in on clouds. Gods were worshiped with pomp. In the time of Jesus Christ, the Roman emperor was considered a god, and his people were expected to burn incense to him in worship.

And yet, here was God himself, condemned by a subordinate of that very emperor to die, and forced to carry a heavy tree limb on his shoulder, through the streets of a city surrounded by crowds. While the emperor enjoyed music and offerings, the God who came to redeem us was weighed down by wood and surrounded by jeering crowds. How did Jesus feel at this moment?

We believe that Jesus told us to love one another as he loved us. With the love of God, the expanseless, total love to which we aspire and which we can only respond with His grace.

Are there people in our nursing lives who are bearing a heavy cross? While half of humanity exalts itself to live like Roman gods, are there workers, patients and families we encounter who are ground down into the dirt?

Faith in action

Do you see someone who is bearing a heavy cross today? Something shameful, heavy or unbearable?

At one time in your life did you exalt ourselves at the cost of diminishing another person? Can you confess this and try to make amends in some small way to that person today?

THE THIRD STATION: JESUS FALLS THE THIRD TIME

We adore you O Christ, and we praise you.

Because by your holy Cross, you have redeemed the world.

It wasn't supposed to be like this.

You may have been a nurse a month, a year or five years before you reached this nadir.

A beloved patient has died.

You did all you could to help this person. You not only tried; you exhausted yourself. That last sip of water or the last kind word represented the point at which you gave your all.

We live in a culture that teaches us trying doesn't count. We brutally assign worth according to consequences and outcomes.

Nurses know better.

As we fall under the weight of the Cross, we know that that "trying" had value.

The first time I encountered a patient death, a chaplain reminded me that we are the midwives helping that person into heaven.

And yet, when a patient's last words to us are, "I love you," we encounter a loss that is too hard to carry. We can only remember that God himself dropped that big heavy cross on the way to Calvary.

To err is human. To fall under the weight of a Cross is divine.

The more you love, the harder that fall is. May it be blessed; may your heart grow larger each time the suffering of others wounds you.

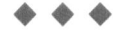

Faith in action

Are there ways that my nursing failures are redemptive? How do they prevent me from operating from a place of pride?

Do the lessons learned, and the heartbreak of loss teach me new things that strengthen my ability to serve?

THE FOURTH STATION: JESUS MEETS HIS AFFLICTED MOTHER

We adore you O Christ, and we praise you.

Because by your holy Cross, you have redeemed the world.

How this "station" conflicts with our present-day values! For in this moment clashed a mother's social shame and her divine faith.

Would we as nurses tell the mother of Jesus that his crime was his own choice, and he needed to accept the consequences of his action? We hope not. Yet we separate mothers from children on the Way of the Cross in other ways. Our lectures about self-care can potentially harm them both.

Do we tell mothers of troubled children that going down into the mess won't save their child, but will only harm them too? Did Mary of Nazareth by chance have a neighbor who told her not to go out that day, to attend to her headache, to spare herself the gory sufferings of her Son's execution? After all, Mary, she could have said, wasn't He the one who decided to tell everyone He was God? It was his agency... his choice...

But Mary believed. Mary taught all Christians, at his first miracle in Cana in Galilee, to "do whatever he tells you." He told her, with those in the crowd, to take up her cross daily and follow Him. Tradition has taught us that she followed him as closely as she could up Calvary hill... even to stand at the foot of his Cross, covered in His blood.

She knew it was not shame to follow Him and endorse Him. She knew that the meaning of the condemnation, which all of Jerusalem cheered that day, was wrong, and that her Son was someone else.

During our walk as nurses, we find ourselves accompanying people who suffer as the result of their choices. Like Mary, our eyes see beyond this. This person is someone else, the child of some mother.... in fact, the creature of the Living God, capable of becoming His adopted child through grace.

Because Christ told us that whatever we do to this person, we do unto Him, we have the permission, and the duty, to do what we can to heal them.

Go in peace today. Heal the addict, the criminal, the glutton, and the filthy one today. Help that heart patient whose family has hidden a McDonald's cheeseburger on the windowsill. It really is okay. They need your help not because they deserve it... but because Christ commanded you to give it.

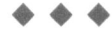

Faith in action

Has your work as a nurse, your willingness to serve at personal cost, ever caused you to be accused of being "codependent"? Do people who try to apply the logic of disease to the nursing profession really understand Matthew 25?

Does the nursing culture in your workplace shun or label certain people or groups of people? Are the drinkers or overeaters or the lawless or disabled seen as less worthy of care? As such, are we straying from the Christian vision of health care as a God-given human right?

THE FIFTH STATION: SIMON OF CYRENE HELPS JESUS CARRY HIS CROSS

We adore you O Christ, and we praise you.

Because by your holy Cross, you have redeemed the world.

It is five o'clock. The alarm clock rings gratingly. You put your head under the pillow in vain, hitting snooze. You do not want to go to work today.

Hopefully you are still the nurse who does not believe in "calling off." Hopefully you keep your word, and still have scruples about upending a schedule at the last minute. Hopefully you still have a problem with mandating the night shift person to stay, or sending someone scrambling for a replacement an hour before you report on.

When you are pressed into service, on days like this, you are like Simon the Cyrenean. In Jerusalem for a lovely Passover, he ended up being forced by Roman soldiers to carry the cross of Jesus.

The Gospel mentions him as the father of Rufus and Alexander, presumably two people known to the early Christians.

His perseverance and life-changing encounter that day was surely the kernel of faith in the lives of Rufus and Alexander, apparently renowned in first-century Christian circles.

Maybe today, at seven a.m., you will have a life changing encounter. Unbeknownst to you, the work you do today may impact your community just as Simon's chance encounter with Jesus impacted Rufus and Alexander.

If you call off today, you will miss that opportunity.

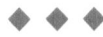

Faith in action

Recall an important relationship you have forged in your life as a nurse or a student. Did this encounter seem significant at the time?
Could you have missed this moment?

THE SIXTH STATION: VERONICA WIPES THE FACE OF JESUS

We adore you O Christ, and we praise you.

Because by your holy Cross, you have redeemed the world.

Western Christian tradition has it that a holy lady in Jerusalem named Veronica took pity on Jesus and brought a cloth over to him to wipe the blood, sweat and spit out of his eyes. Tradition has it that God thanked her by imprinting his face on her cloth. The veil of Veronica is kept to this day.

While this was one of the traditions edited out by the Reformation Christians, it is a powerful story for nurses.

When we bathe a patient, or wipe their face with a washcloth, or change a brief, is it possible that God—who says whatever we do to these least ones, we do to Him—might imprint his face on that washcloth? In the Kingdom of Heaven, will we be presented by angels with all these washcloths, along with a thank you note from God, remembering every act of kindness done to a fellow traveler in our nursing life?

What if these small acts mean so much? Isn't that what Jesus taught us?

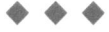

Faith in action

Instead of delegating all the bathing to nursing assistants today, wash at least one patient's face, remembering to do so with reverence and gentleness.

THE SEVENTH STATION: JESUS FALLS THE SECOND TIME

We adore you O Christ, and we praise you.

Because by your holy Cross, you have redeemed the world.

In Catholic grade school, did the children ever think Jesus was clumsy? How could he fall so many times on such a short walk? Superman wouldn't have fallen once.

Why would tradition teach us that Jesus Christ would fall under the weight of the Cross not just once, but three times? Was this traditional belief mistaken? Could the God who walked on water really fall?

Wasn't his faith great enough to save him?

But isn't this similar to what the crowds said when they mocked him: He saved others, but himself he cannot save. If he is God, let him come down from that Cross.

Hence, the tradition that the God who willingly let himself be fastened to a tree would also allow himself to become exhausted under its weight.

As nurses we can see ourselves as the superheroes on the unit… the deus ex machina who arrives on the scene when someone is supine and helpless. "Hello, my name is…. I'll be your nurse today," we begin, and all is meant to create an angelic illusion of safety.

We represent the divine, not necessarily for God, but for the corporations. It's called customer service.

Today, are you clumsy like Jesus? Are you allowed to be human as you walk alongside your patients, or are you a doll in a uniform performing customer service? Did you know it's okay to be human today?

◆ ◆ ◆

Faith in action

Give up the perfectionism and acknowledge your mistakes or lack of knowledge today.

Ask a supervisor a question about something you don't know.

THE EIGHTH STATION: JESUS SPEAKS TO THE WOMEN OF JERUSALEM

We adore you O Christ, and we praise you.

Because by your holy Cross, you have redeemed the world.

"Weep not for me, but weep for yourselves and your children." Shocking words from a man about to die. How bad could it get for the women of Jerusalem? In 70 A.D., they found out. The Arch of Titus in Rome commemorates the sad procession of Jewish slaves, dragged through the streets of Rome with their menorahs and their children, after the destruction of the temple and the city.

How many times will we hear someone say to us, "I don't know what anyone would want to do your job. I could never do it. Why would you want to help us go to the bathroom, or feed us, or see all the things you do?"

Yes, we suffer on the job. Some days, we suffer a lot.

Yet, weep not for me, you say with Jesus.

Because the strength from working as a nurse far outweighs the challenges. We are rarely bored, and we rarely come home from work feeling we have accomplished nothing. We can look back on a year and see that it is so full that one year is like seven. One decade of nursing life is like a generation.

Weep not for the nurse, with her modest wages, ugly uniforms, and curtailed social life.

Weep for those who do not know that it is the common job of humanity to care for the sick and the weak.

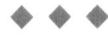

Faith in action

Think of, and rejoice in, one hidden benefit of your life as a nurse. Thank God for this upside, no matter how small or hidden it is.

Give up the pity parties about mandating, workplace drama and office politics today.

THE NINTH STATION: JESUS FALLS THE THIRD TIME

We adore you O Christ, and we praise you.

Because by your holy Cross, you have redeemed the world.

Again? Why this final fall?

Isn't it a reminder that, as mortality approaches, the dying are frail, and more likely to fall?

Jesus' Morse Fall Scale rating would have been off the charts. He had endured previous falls, had been injured, had environmental hazards in his way, and had lost a great deal of blood. His vision and hearing were probably impaired, and he was most likely not wearing nonskid footwear.

All of these fall risks occured by design, as the torments were part of his execution even before he went to the cross.

Here are two realities: frailty and torture.

Maybe you have witnessed the two together in the gunshot victims in your Emergency Department. Or as you held the hand of a dying client who endures the torment of not having visitors. Violence and neglect stalk the weak.

But today you are called to alleviate the ailment as well as the torment.

◆ ◆ ◆

Faith in action

How can I be an advocate for the weakest person I see today?

How can I advocate for people in my personal life, without violating professional boundaries? Can I donate band-aids to a charity, bring dinner to an ailing neighbor, or serve as a voice for the voiceless?

THE TENTH STATION: JESUS IS STRIPPED OF HIS GARMENTS

We adore you O Christ, and we praise you.

Because by your holy Cross, you have redeemed the world.

This station commemorates the humiliations of Jesus.

Suffering not only encompasses pain, but also humiliation.

There is the helplessness of the post-surgical client who is unable to walk. The new mother who is giving up her baby for adoption, experiencing disenfranchised grief. The mother who walks into your WIC clinic, admitting to you and the community that she does not have the wherewithal to feed a family.

It is hard to accept help.

How can you affirm the client's dignity today even as you offer them your help?

◆ ◆ ◆

Faith in action

Where in your community do altered health status and stigma go hand in hand? Poverty? HIV/AIDS? Opiod addiction?

Research your state's public health goals and become aware of the psychological and emotional impact of compromised health status.

THE ELEVENTH STATION: JESUS IS NAILED TO THE CROSS

We adore you O Christ, and we praise you.
Because by your holy Cross, you have redeemed the world.

There was no turning back. Jesus, fully God, was also fully human, and was tempted. Perhaps, up till now, Jesus fought a temptation to go back to Pilate and negotiate. Now, as he was fastened to the Cross, the decision to love and offer himself for our salvation was irrevocable.

The day also came when you realized there was no turning back from nursing.

Perhaps it was the day your first student loan bill arrived.

Perhaps it came sooner, with an inner conviction you couldn't shake.

The commitment, at some point, became real. It was a moment of pride, joy, and probably panic. The feeling of being in too deep accompanied by the rational conclusion that in fact you were in too deep to turn back now.

Jesus' horrible moment of truth gave us a God who truly sympathizes with our weakness and panic when we feel we are in over our heads.

He knows what it is like. He took that pain on, so that giving so freely to others would become a source of Life and Triumph and resurrection.

◆ ◆ ◆

Faith in action

Review your current career commitments, and prior life commitments. Is there a God-honoring prior commitment that has given way to careerism?

How can you streamline your time management to balance your prior commitments and your nursing calling?

THE TWELFTH STATION: JESUS DIES ON THE CROSS

We adore you O Christ, and we praise you.

Because by your holy Cross, you have redeemed the world.

One of the privileges and burdens of our calling is that we can stand with John, the Mother of Jesus, and Mary Magdalen at the foot of the Cross.

How hard it is. We weep, comfort, and encourage. We focus on the real, happy meaning of the transition and help the person go there in peace.

We grieve a special kind of grief, one that is hidden behind our efforts to minister to patients and families. Without frequent debriefing, we can become traumatized by our constant walk through the shadow of death. Or we can grow cold.

Can you trust God to reward you for all this hidden pain? Does he not see your constant watch at the bedsides of others? Can you trust him to provide kindness, wisdom and inspiration for that time when you are eighty-five or ninety and need someone to be there for you?

He has been there. And you have been there for others. Trust him with your mortality. He has already been there and is preparing a reward and a blessed passage for you.

Faith in action

If you only had another six months to live, what would you do today?

Rather than put these things off, can you do them anyway today?

Dive into your bucket list. Brainstorm and add fifty items to it today. Live the gift each day.

THE THIRTEENTH STATION: JESUS IS TAKEN DOWN FROM THE CROSS

We adore you O Christ, and we praise you.

Because by your holy Cross, you have redeemed the world.

Some doctors and nurses find closure in funerals. Others avoid them.

Yet, we all need a burial ritual for our own peace of mind. One nurse clips obituaries from the paper, building an album full of the names and stories of the patients she has helped.

During that personal moment when family and friends release the loved one from the Cross, where can you be found? Are you interceding for them? Sending a card? Or hiding?

If you are hiding, could it be that you are still coping with another personal loss?

Can you heal today, from the death of a grandparent, friend, favorite patient or role model? Do you not know that today He is risen, and you do not need to remain on that cross?

Faith in action

Today, go to God and ask Him to heal the grief in your heart, from lost loved ones, broken dreams, or strained relationships.

Think of the care plan you would design for the grieving nurse and be kind enough to do these things for yourself today.

THE FOURTEENTH STATION: JESUS IS LAID IN THE TOMB

We adore you O Christ, and we praise you.

Because by your holy Cross, you have redeemed the world.

He had nowhere to lay his head and was a homeless itinerant preacher.

A wealthy man named Joseph honored him and gave him his own tomb.

There are times when our nursing lives give us the opportunity to enhance a person's dignity at a key moment.

We help them get funding for badly needed psychiatric medications. We dig into our own pockets to buy them new shirts to replace the stained ones they wear and cannot see because of failing eyesight. We realize someone cannot read and go the extra mile to encourage them to seek out the literacy council.

These decisions change a life, a family tree, the future of a nation.

Joseph's decision to give up his tomb to bury the itinerant preacher from Nazareth changed the course of history.

How could Jesus be raised from the tomb, if no one had offered him one?

What extra nursing intervention seems small to you, but could change the course of history today?

◆ ◆ ◆

Faith in action

When you meet the next client, think beyond the usual reference to a primary care physician.

What wrap around resources, specialist appointments, and work/life balance issues could change this person's life, and impact the future?

THE FIFTEENTH STATION: JESUS RISES FROM THE DEAD

We adore you O Christ, and we praise you.

Because by your holy Cross, you have redeemed the world.

As a popular Christian song says, "The Cross meant to kill is my victory." The logic of the Cross is that the very thing meant to destroy Jesus, His death, was the means of His triumph.

The workdays that exhaust my physical, mental and emotional resources are usually my best days.

Where I have gone beyond myself and am giving 110% but 120% is demanded… the day does not destroy me. Somehow it leads to excellence and higher outcomes.

Can you think of a day when the very thing meant to destroy you--- a hostile family, a real-life tornado or fire, or an unexpected code—turned out to be your finest hour?

This triumph over destructive forces is what we call "Glory."

It is Resurrection power released in your life by God's grace.

Take a time to savor the glory of your nursing journey today.

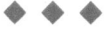

Faith in action

Create a "glory journal" for your nursing journey.

Catalogue those moments when you felt you were going under, only to rise above the waves to new heights.

Let every page be filled with thankfulness.

www.ingramcontent.com/pod-product-compliance
Lightning Source LLC
Chambersburg PA
CBHW030011190526
45157CB00015B/2404